Headache Tracker

MONTHLY TOTAL

MONTH

MONDAY	TUESDAY	WEDNESDAY	THURSDAY	FRIDAY	SATURDAY	SUNDAY

DATE

DURATION

INTENSITY

PAIN CHARACTERISTICS

TREATMENT

WHERE IT HURTS

FACTORS

SLEEP

CAFFEINE

ALCOHOL

WATER

FOOD

WEATHER

OTHER FACTORS

NOTES

DATE

DURATION

INTENSITY

PAIN CHARACTERISTICS

TREATMENT

WHERE IT HURTS

FACTORS

SLEEP

CAFFEINE

ALCOHOL

WATER

FOOD

WEATHER

OTHER FACTORS

NOTES

DATE

DURATION

INTENSITY

PAIN CHARACTERISTICS

TREATMENT

WHERE IT HURTS

FACTORS

SLEEP

CAFFEINE

ALCOHOL

WATER

FOOD

WEATHER

OTHER FACTORS

NOTES

DATE
DURATION
INTENSITY
PAIN CHARACTERISTICS
TREATMENT
WHERE IT HURTS
FACTORS
SLEEP
CAFFEINE
ALCOHOL
WATER
FOOD
WEATHER
OTHER FACTORS
NOTES

DATE

DURATION

INTENSITY

PAIN CHARACTERISTICS

TREATMENT

WHERE IT HURTS

FACTORS

SLEEP

CAFFEINE

ALCOHOL

WATER

FOOD

WEATHER

OTHER FACTORS

NOTES

DATE

DURATION

INTENSITY

PAIN CHARACTERISTICS

TREATMENT

WHERE IT HURTS

FACTORS

SLEEP

CAFFEINE

ALCOHOL

WATER

FOOD

WEATHER

OTHER FACTORS

NOTES

DATE

DURATION

INTENSITY

PAIN CHARACTERISTICS

TREATMENT

WHERE IT HURTS

FACTORS

SLEEP

CAFFEINE

ALCOHOL

WATER

FOOD

WEATHER

OTHER FACTORS

NOTES

DATE

DURATION

INTENSITY

PAIN CHARACTERISTICS

TREATMENT

WHERE IT HURTS

FACTORS

SLEEP

CAFFEINE

ALCOHOL

WATER

FOOD

WEATHER

OTHER FACTORS

NOTES

DATE

DURATION

INTENSITY

PAIN CHARACTERISTICS

TREATMENT

WHERE IT HURTS

FACTORS

SLEEP

CAFFEINE

ALCOHOL

WATER

FOOD

WEATHER

OTHER FACTORS

NOTES

DATE

DURATION

INTENSITY

PAIN CHARACTERISTICS

TREATMENT

WHERE IT HURTS

FACTORS

SLEEP

OTHER FACTORS

CAFFEINE

ALCOHOL

WATER

FOOD

WEATHER

NOTES

DATE

DURATION

INTENSITY

PAIN CHARACTERISTICS

TREATMENT

WHERE IT HURTS

FACTORS

SLEEP

CAFFEINE

ALCOHOL

WATER

FOOD

WEATHER

OTHER FACTORS

NOTES

DATE

DURATION

INTENSITY

PAIN CHARACTERISTICS

TREATMENT

WHERE IT HURTS

FACTORS

SLEEP

OTHER FACTORS

CAFFEINE

ALCOHOL

WATER

FOOD

WEATHER

NOTES

DATE

DURATION

INTENSITY

PAIN CHARACTERISTICS

TREATMENT

WHERE IT HURTS

FACTORS

SLEEP

OTHER FACTORS

CAFFEINE

ALCOHOL

WATER

FOOD

WEATHER

NOTES

DATE

DURATION

INTENSITY

PAIN CHARACTERISTICS

TREATMENT

FACTORS

SLEEP

CAFFEINE

ALCOHOL

WATER

FOOD

WEATHER

OTHER FACTORS

NOTES

DATE

DURATION

INTENSITY

PAIN CHARACTERISTICS

TREATMENT

WHERE IT HURTS

FACTORS

SLEEP

CAFFEINE

ALCOHOL

WATER

FOOD

WEATHER

OTHER FACTORS

NOTES

DATE

DURATION

INTENSITY

PAIN CHARACTERISTICS

TREATMENT

WHERE IT HURTS

FACTORS

SLEEP

CAFFEINE

ALCOHOL

WATER

FOOD

WEATHER

OTHER FACTORS

NOTES

FACTORS

SLEEP

CAFFEINE

ALCOHOL

WATER

FOOD

WEATHER

OTHER FACTORS

NOTES

DATE

DURATION

WHERE IT HURTS

INTENSITY

PAIN CHARACTERISTICS

TREATMENT

FACTORS

SLEEP

CAFFEINE

ALCOHOL

WATER

FOOD

WEATHER

OTHER FACTORS

NOTES

DATE

DURATION

INTENSITY

PAIN CHARACTERISTICS

TREATMENT

WHERE IT HURTS

FACTORS

SLEEP

CAFFEINE

ALCOHOL

WATER

FOOD

WEATHER

OTHER FACTORS

NOTES

DATE

DURATION

INTENSITY

PAIN CHARACTERISTICS

TREATMENT

WHERE IT HURTS

FACTORS

SLEEP

CAFFEINE

ALCOHOL

WATER

FOOD

WEATHER

OTHER FACTORS

NOTES

DATE_________________________

DURATION_________________________

INTENSITY

PAIN CHARACTERISTICS

TREATMENT

WHERE IT HURTS

FACTORS

SLEEP

CAFFEINE

ALCOHOL

WATER

FOOD

WEATHER

OTHER FACTORS

NOTES

DATE

DURATION

WHERE IT HURTS

INTENSITY

PAIN CHARACTERISTICS

TREATMENT

FACTORS

SLEEP

CAFFEINE

ALCOHOL

WATER

FOOD

WEATHER

OTHER FACTORS

NOTES

WHERE IT HURTS

FACTORS

SLEEP

CAFFEINE

ALCOHOL

WATER

FOOD

WEATHER

OTHER FACTORS

NOTES

DATE

DURATION

INTENSITY

PAIN CHARACTERISTICS

TREATMENT

WHERE IT HURTS

FACTORS

SLEEP

CAFFEINE

ALCOHOL

WATER

FOOD

WEATHER

OTHER FACTORS

NOTES

DATE

DURATION

INTENSITY

PAIN CHARACTERISTICS

TREATMENT

WHERE IT HURTS

FACTORS

SLEEP

CAFFEINE

ALCOHOL

WATER

FOOD

WEATHER

OTHER FACTORS

NOTES

DATE_______________

DURATION_______________

WHERE IT HURTS

INTENSITY

PAIN CHARACTERISTICS

TREATMENT

FACTORS

SLEEP

CAFFEINE

ALCOHOL

WATER

FOOD

WEATHER

OTHER FACTORS

NOTES

DATE

DURATION

INTENSITY

PAIN CHARACTERISTICS

TREATMENT

WHERE IT HURTS

FACTORS

SLEEP

CAFFEINE

ALCOHOL

WATER

FOOD

WEATHER

OTHER FACTORS

NOTES

DATE
DURATION
INTENSITY
PAIN CHARACTERISTICS
TREATMENT
WHERE IT HURTS
FACTORS
SLEEP
CAFFEINE
ALCOHOL
WATER
FOOD
WEATHER
OTHER FACTORS
NOTES

DATE

DURATION

INTENSITY

PAIN CHARACTERISTICS

TREATMENT

WHERE IT HURTS

FACTORS

SLEEP

OTHER FACTORS

CAFFEINE

ALCOHOL

WATER

FOOD

WEATHER

NOTES

DATE

DURATION

INTENSITY

PAIN CHARACTERISTICS

TREATMENT

WHERE IT HURTS

FACTORS

SLEEP

CAFFEINE

ALCOHOL

WATER

FOOD

WEATHER

OTHER FACTORS

NOTES

DATE

DURATION

INTENSITY

PAIN CHARACTERISTICS

TREATMENT

WHERE IT HURTS

FACTORS

SLEEP

CAFFEINE

ALCOHOL

WATER

FOOD

WEATHER

OTHER FACTORS

NOTES

DATE

DURATION

INTENSITY

PAIN CHARACTERISTICS

TREATMENT

WHERE IT HURTS

FACTORS

SLEEP

CAFFEINE

ALCOHOL

WATER

FOOD

WEATHER

OTHER FACTORS

NOTES

DATE

DURATION

INTENSITY

PAIN CHARACTERISTICS

TREATMENT

FACTORS

SLEEP

CAFFEINE

ALCOHOL

WATER

FOOD

WEATHER

OTHER FACTORS

NOTES

DATE

DURATION

INTENSITY

PAIN CHARACTERISTICS

TREATMENT

WHERE IT HURTS

FACTORS

SLEEP

CAFFEINE

ALCOHOL

WATER

FOOD

WEATHER

OTHER FACTORS

NOTES

DATE

DURATION

INTENSITY

PAIN CHARACTERISTICS

TREATMENT

WHERE IT HURTS

FACTORS

SLEEP

CAFFEINE

ALCOHOL

WATER

FOOD

WEATHER

OTHER FACTORS

NOTES

DATE_____________________

DURATION_____________________

INTENSITY

PAIN CHARACTERISTICS

TREATMENT

WHERE IT HURTS

FACTORS

SLEEP

CAFFEINE

ALCOHOL

WATER

FOOD

WEATHER

OTHER FACTORS

NOTES

DATE_______________________

DURATION___________________

WHERE IT HURTS

INTENSITY

PAIN CHARACTERISTICS

TREATMENT

FACTORS

SLEEP

CAFFEINE

ALCOHOL

WATER

FOOD

WEATHER

OTHER FACTORS

NOTES

DATE________________________

DURATION____________________________

WHERE IT HURTS

INTENSITY

PAIN CHARACTERISTICS

TREATMENT

FACTORS

SLEEP

CAFFEINE

ALCOHOL

WATER

FOOD

WEATHER

OTHER FACTORS

NOTES

FACTORS

SLEEP

CAFFEINE

ALCOHOL

WATER

FOOD

WEATHER

OTHER FACTORS

NOTES

DATE

DURATION

INTENSITY

PAIN CHARACTERISTICS

TREATMENT

WHERE IT HURTS

FACTORS

SLEEP

OTHER FACTORS

CAFFEINE

ALCOHOL

WATER

FOOD

WEATHER

NOTES

DATE

DURATION

WHERE IT HURTS

INTENSITY

PAIN CHARACTERISTICS

TREATMENT

FACTORS

SLEEP

CAFFEINE

ALCOHOL

WATER

FOOD

WEATHER

OTHER FACTORS

NOTES

DATE______________________________   DURATION________________

WHERE IT HURTS

INTENSITY

PAIN CHARACTERISTICS

TREATMENT

FACTORS

SLEEP

CAFFEINE

ALCOHOL

WATER

FOOD

WEATHER

OTHER FACTORS

NOTES

DATE

DURATION

INTENSITY

PAIN CHARACTERISTICS

TREATMENT

WHERE IT HURTS

FACTORS

SLEEP

CAFFEINE

ALCOHOL

WATER

FOOD

WEATHER

OTHER FACTORS

NOTES

WHERE IT HURTS

FACTORS

SLEEP

CAFFEINE

ALCOHOL

WATER

FOOD

WEATHER

OTHER FACTORS

NOTES

DATE________________

DURATION________________

INTENSITY

PAIN CHARACTERISTICS

TREATMENT

WHERE IT HURTS

FACTORS

SLEEP

CAFFEINE

ALCOHOL

WATER

FOOD

WEATHER

OTHER FACTORS

NOTES

DATE

DURATION

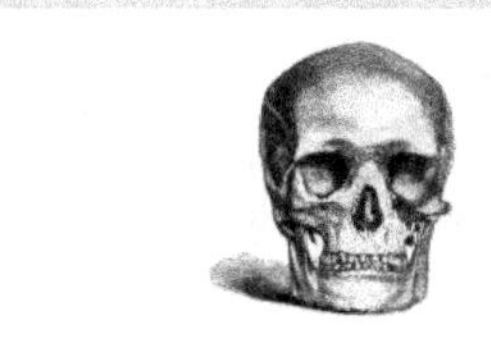

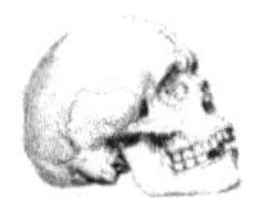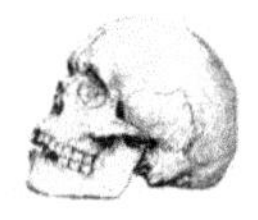

WHERE IT HURTS

INTENSITY

PAIN CHARACTERISTICS

TREATMENT

FACTORS

SLEEP

CAFFEINE

ALCOHOL

WATER

FOOD

WEATHER

OTHER FACTORS

NOTES

INTENSITY

PAIN CHARACTERISTICS

TREATMENT

FACTORS

SLEEP

OTHER FACTORS

CAFFEINE

ALCOHOL

WATER

FOOD

WEATHER

NOTES